The Clear Skin Solution:

Overcoming Eczema and Psoriasis for Infants through Adults

JOLIE McSHANE, INHC

ISBN: 9781733692618

CONTENTS

INTRODUCTION

How did I end up here—back in school in my 50s, writing a book about eczema? My relentless questioning frustrated doctors who couldn't give me clear answers about the root cause of this condition. I refused to accept vague explanations or the standard pill-for-every-ill approach of our medical system. That determination left me standing alone, but it also led me to uncover life-changing insights.

I wrote this book for the moms who, like me, are exhausted by dead-end treatments and desperate for real solutions. Some doctors may have thought I was nuts, but if advocating for health makes me a "health nut," then I wear that label with pride—because that mindset saved lives, including my son's.

The American health system is desperate for reform. A shift in focus from medical care to health care would profoundly improve the resilience of a society addicted to prescription drugs. We need more focus on health care and less on medical care. Please understand, if I am in a car accident, the first person I want to see is a medical doctor. However, medical doctors are not trained to handle the chronic illnesses caused by our country's poor dietary habits and high levels of toxins in our foods. Toxins that the FDA, USDA, NIH and CDC allow to exist since their definition is Generally Recognized As Safe (GRAS) for thousands of chemicals added to our foods.

Having always been interested in health, nutrition books were my sole source of pleasure reading. Enrolling in a nutrition school (Institute for

Integrative Nutrition) opened my eyes to a new world of healthy foods and outstanding dietary theories. Part of the education was to learn about my own health journey and understand the finer details of health histories. It was during this part of my education that I realized why my children were diagnosed with ADHD, ear infections, sleepwalking, allergies, frequent childhood illnesses, and later depression. The birth of my third child late in life changed everything.

My son was allergic in vitro, every time I consumed milk products, the fetus would violently toss and turn for hours. I immediately eliminated milk and milk products during my pregnancy. After his birth at three months of age, we noticed his skin would break out in red bumps and rashes. By 5 months, he had total body coverage of eczema. No one slept—neither the baby, who would fuss all night trying to scratch, nor the parents, who had to keep vigil to prevent him from tearing holes in his skin. Every morning, he woke up with blood covered sheets.

His pediatrician never examined him. We were at a standoff. The doctor refused to lay eyes on him unless he was immunized, and I would not immunize him, fearing that the additional toxins in his system would worsen his eczema. (These were pre-internet days, so I was totally on my own. We now know that if we had immunized him, his eczema would have become life-threatening. If hospitalized, the open wounds invite staph infections, and he would have been knocking on death's door.)

I then pursued a desperate hunt for someone who could help us. I greatly appreciated those professionals who admitted they could not help. The professionals who wrote prescriptions for cortisone cream were merely covering up the problem. As many of you know, long-term use of cortisone cream thins the skin and damages the liver. This was not a solution; it was simply a band-aid. Putting these creams on a 5-month-old child is not acceptable.

Living in Baltimore next to one of the best hospitals in the world, Johns Hopkins, I found a pediatric dermatologist. Sadly, his advice was nonsense. Smothering the child in Vaseline turned out to be one of the worst nights of his life. Now I understand why—the toxins were locked into his body with no way to escape. Thankfully, my son has no recollection of this event.

The pediatric allergist couldn't help either. My son tested positive for allergies to almost everything. I received the "Dust Mite" theory and was given a catalog of recommended products to eliminate dust mites from his room. My advice? Please don't waste your money! Dust mites thrive between 65-75 degrees and die otherwise. Just open the windows daily and let the room air out (this has been a common practice in Europe, where they place bedding on the windowsill for the day).

The Johns Hopkins pediatric environmental allergist, pediatrician, and nutritionist offered little support, leaving me to navigate on my own. Desperate, I traveled to the National Institutes of Health in Washington, DC, the world's largest medical library. I hoped to find answers but left empty-handed, except for references to potential vitamin deficiencies like B-vitamins, Vitamin D, fish oils, and a brief mention of Leaky Gut Syndrome. Could this be the key? Is there a connection between leaky gut, eczema, and digestion? Maybe a Pediatric Gastroenterologist could provide some answers.

Fortunately, a pediatric gastroenterologist named Dr. Alan Lake resided in Baltimore, just down the street. I prayed that he would have the solution. As I awaited the appointment, belief in my discovery grew stronger. Food played a crucial role in my son's good and bad days. Which foods would ease his symptoms? What could I feed him? Dr. Alan Lake confirmed my son's condition as leaky gut syndrome and prescribed a special hypo-allergenic formula, restricting his diet to jarred commercial baby foods like peaches, peas, and baby rice. We were warned that his condition might worsen before the formula was accepted by his body. Despite the challenges, we persevered, avoiding hospitalization where open wounds and staph infection could lead to death. The 60th hour was the most difficult, but he made it through.

We had overcome the worst part of this ordeal, and my son's eczema started to clear up. By the age of 1, he could consume four foods (hypoallergenic formula, baby rice, peaches and pears). By the age of 2 he expanded to 10 foods. We thought things were improving, but then asthma struck. It was far worse than eczema, life-threatening on many occasions. Eczema, allergies, and asthma were all interconnected, stemming from leaky gut syndrome. Healing the gut meant gaining control over eczema, asthma, and allergies... forever!

The journey continued for another 10 years, seeking a plethora of professionals, experts, alternative health care practitioners, and making dietary changes. The beautiful life-changing epiphanies occurred when I returned to school and enrolled in the Institute for Integrative Nutrition, studying over 50 dietary theories. The dietary theory that aligned with my family's health goals was Dr. Weston Price and the Weston A. Price Foundation. Combining those theories with Dr. Natasha Campbell-McBride's GAPS Diet completed the puzzle. I was once told that my son would never grow past four feet tall and likely die by age 7. Instead, I have a happy, handsome, successful 27-year-old son who brings smiles, love and contributes to society. He leads a healthy, normal life, free from asthma and eczema, with only a few remaining allergies including peanuts, shellfish, and pasteurized milk products (raw milk is fine).

After a gut-wrenching decade dedicated to sleepless nights spent reading health books to heal my son, I have dedicated much of my life helping other moms facing similar struggles with their babies. The secret is simple, it's as simple as food, good food!

Here I am now, wanting to share my knowledge and spare other families the pain of living with these conditions. Babies heal rapidly; their bodies possess remarkable restorative powers. A one-year-old client with severe eczema healed within 1 ½ months, while a seven-year-old was healed within 3 months. Adults (unfortunately) take longer, but they do see improvements within two weeks of starting the regimen.

"Health is Wealth" is my motto. By eating healthy, you'll feel better, have more energy, accomplish more, maintain a positive attitude, and live a fulfilling life. If only I had known, then what I know now.

1

BY THE NUMBERS: UNRAVELING THE TRUTH

Let me hit you with some eye-opening facts; 20-25% of patients who walk through the doors of dermatologists are eczema or psoriasis sufferers. It doesn't discriminate between men and women, it's an equal-opportunity tormentor. When does it like to strike? Right from the get-go; infancy and childhood are its favorite hunting grounds.

Here's the sad truth, there is no medically documented cause for eczema or psoriasis. A staggering 65% of sufferers start experiencing those pesky symptoms in their very first year of life. And 85%? Well, they're in for a bumpy ride before they even reach the age of 5. And those living in concrete jungles and dry, unforgiving climates are more likely to bear the brunt of this condition. Even in adulthood, we're looking at a prevalence rate of around 7%.

How much does this cost our society? In the United States, atopic dermatitis costs each patient an average of $600 a year. Doctor visits, medication, over-the-counter remedies, lubricants, and days lost from work—they all add up. When you tally it all up for the entire US population, we're looking at a mind-boggling $5 billion a year.

However, experts at the National Institutes of Health claim there's no established cure for eczema and psoriasis. I beg to differ and this book will provide you with healing solutions.

If you want to dig deeper into the numbers listed above, check out the source: National Institutes for Health (https://pubmed.ncbi.nlm.nih.gov/29063433/).

2

THE ECZEMA FREE PLAN: HOW DO WE ACHIEVE FREEDOM FROM ECZEMA?

#1 – Acknowledge the correlation between diet, eczema / psoriasis and digestive inflammation. This is the number one hurdle to surpass to move toward healing.

What? Really? Why has my doctor never discussed this with me? Sadly, the connection between digestive health and skin problems is not widely acknowledged in mainstream medicine. However, a few medical professionals are now providing information to help eczema/psoriasis sufferers understand the link between digestive health and this chronic condition. Check out the list of medical professionals below and visit their websites for more detailed information.

Gut and Psychology Syndrome – Dr. Natasha Campbell-McBride, MD (www.gaps.com)

Ultra-Prevention - Dr. Mark Hyman – www.drmarkhyman.com

Healing the New Childhood Epidemics – Dr. Kenneth Bock and Cameron Stauth

The Gut Balance Revolution – Dr. Gerard Mullin

The Gut Repair Cookbook – Dr. Josh Axe

Dr. William Davis – Super Gut

Dr. Casey Means – Good Energy

Eczema and psoriasis have very little to do with your skin and everything to do with your digestive tract. Your body is simply trying to communicate that something is wrong on the inside by exhibiting symptoms on the outside. This kind of communication from the body happens all the time. When we're cold, the body sends a message to the brain: "You're cold, get warm!" A fever can indicate an infection, virus, or cold. So why should eczema be any different?

Recent research refers to the digestive system as the "second brain," this makes sense. The digestive system is where food is processed and broken down to provide nourishment and replenish fluids throughout the body. According to Dr. Michael D. Gershon, author of "The Second Brain" and chairman of the department of anatomy and cell biology at Columbia University, the second brain consists of over 100 million neurons lining the stomach and gut. Fortunately, we don't need to rely on the brain in our heads to digest food; otherwise, we'd be mentally exhausted after every meal!

You know your mental capacity is not as sharp with a lack of sleep, the same holds true with a poor diet. An excellent example of this is feeding a child cake versus whole food. The child's behavior is always modified after consuming sugary nutrition less food. I remember a kindergarten teacher holding birthday parties 15 minutes before the children were released for the day. She had no desire to manage their behavior after eating cupcakes and donuts!

Dr. Natasha McBride's book, "Gut and Psychology Syndrome" (GAPS), delves into extensive research on the relationship between the second brain and how we can heal various ailments by addressing the digestive system. Her remarkable work with autistic children, implementing a diet that heals the gut and significantly improves their symptoms, serves as proof of her success. The book "GAPS Stories: Personal Accounts of Improvement and Recovery Through the GAPS Nutritional Protocol" by Medinform Publishing compiles inspiring testimonials from individuals who have experienced positive results with the GAPS diet.

Achieving freedom from eczema begins with acknowledging that this condition is not merely skin-deep but deeply connected to digestive health. The path to healing lies in understanding the critical role the gut plays in overall wellness and taking intentional steps to address the root causes of inflammation and imbalance. By exploring dietary changes, you can transform your gut, and ultimately, your skin. Remember, eczema is your body's way of communicating that something needs attention—listen to it, nourish it, and empower yourself to take charge of your health. Your journey to being eczema-free starts today.

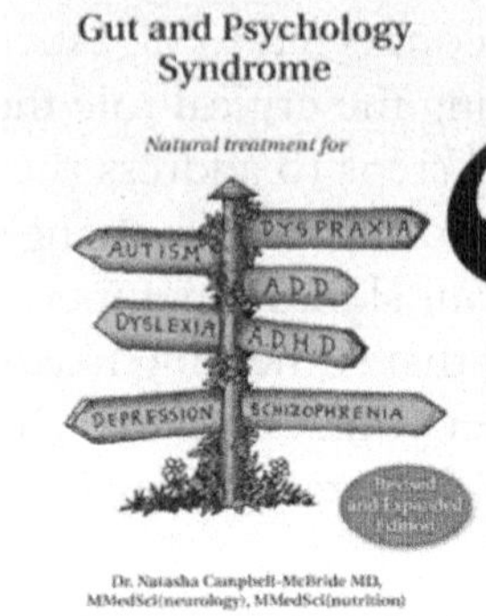

"CHILDREN WHO SUFFER SEVERE ECZEMA IN INFANCY OFTEN DEVELOP AUTISTIC FEATURES LATER IN LIFE

GAPS PATIENTS HAVE BEEN EXPOSED TO NUMBEROUS COURSES OF ANTIBIOTICS

I HAVE YET TO MEET A CHILD WITH AUTISM, ADHD / ADD, ASTHMA, ECZEMA, ALLERGIES, DYSPRAXIA OR DYSLEXIA WHO DOES NOT HAVE DIGESTIVE ABNORMALITIES"

Dr. Natasha Campbell-McBride, MD

3

CAUSES OF ECZEMA & PSORIASIS

There is no single cause of eczema and psoriasis, just as there is no single cause of cancer. The premise of this book is that gut dysbiosis exacerbates all types of eczema, and every individual with eczema suffers from leaky gut syndrome. Therefore, making dietary changes to eliminate harmful foods and introducing healing foods will make a tremendous difference in the lives of all eczema and psoriasis sufferers

WebMD

What is Gut Dysbiosis?

In your gut, there are trillions of microorganisms that make up your gut microbiome. Your gastrointestinal (GI) tract is home to many bacteria, fungi, and viruses... All of these microorganisms keep your gut healthy. When they're out of balance, dysbiosis happens.

How Does Dysbiosis Happen?

When your gut health gets imbalanced and dysbiosis happens, you're more likely to have stomach and other health conditions.

DWebMD - Search What is Gut Dysbiosis

Medical journals have identified potential causes of eczema, including stress, medications, poor diet, and zinc deficiency. However, in every case, internal inflammation accompanies eczema/psoriasis as the body becomes imbalanced due to yeast overgrowth, harmful bacteria, and/or parasites. Individuals with eczema often develop a long list of food sensitivities, which tend to expand over time. This vicious cycle leads to mental imbalance in the form of depression due to the body's inability to absorb nutrients and tolerate fewer foods. This lack of nutritional absorption is referred to as the "gut brain connection" or "gut brain axis".

The terms gut dysbiosis, internal inflammation, gut microbiome disruption and leaky gut syndrome (more in the next chapter) are all similar terms and basically refer to an impaired immune system. Stepping back to look at the big picture, how does the digestive tract become inflamed or leaky? What external factors contribute to eczema? The answer varies from person to person, but the top causes of leaky gut are antibiotics, medications, and the Standard American Diet (SAD).

I truly believe my son's health issues stemmed from a course of antibiotics during my pregnancy, most likely my gut was already inflamed, and the antibiotics wreaked havoc for him in utero.

Over the counter and prescription medications are well documented sources of gut microbiome disruption. Add in a diet with pesticide laden processed foods and our guts become inflamed. We pass our gut biome on to the next generation and unfortunately see exacerbated issues as the next generation struggles with health issues.

Read the full study titled: **The Influence of Nonsteroidal Anti-Inflammatory Drugs on the Gut Microbiome** Source: https://www.ncbi.nlm.nih.gov/pmc/articles/PMC4754147/

Since the 1950s, commercial industrialization of food has become a major industry. Local farms that once served a specific region were transformed into mass producers for the entire nation. This growth in agribusiness also led to the rise of chemical companies, aiding farmers in cultivating high-yielding crops. While this resulted in increased food supply for a growing population, it also introduced thousands of synthetic chemicals and herbicides since the 1950s. The quality of soil has declined, consequently affecting the nutrient content of our food. The Standard American Diet (SAD) has been progressively deteriorating, with more pesticides, additives, preservatives, natural flavors, artificial sugars and highly processed foods causing a rising number of Americans experiencing health issues.

Americans are exposing themselves to a toxic soup of chemically laden foods, exposing our bodies to toxic creams/lotions/hair dye/sunblock and then add in prescription meds. The USDA is allowing over 30 chemical substances that Europeans have banned.

When visiting the doctor, there is very little discussion of diet, nutrient dense foods and healing modalities beyond a pill. As we all witnessed during the Covid pandemic, sadly Americans have the weakest immune systems compared to other 1st world countries.

4

WHAT IS LEAKY GUT SYNDROME?

As discussed in the previous section, eczema or psoriasis is merely a symptom of a damaged digestive system. The term associated with this condition is called leaky gut syndrome.

Leaky Gut Syndrome refers to the condition of "Hyperpermeable Intestines." It means that the lining of the intestines has become porous, with larger and more numerous holes, and the screening process is no longer functioning properly. As a result, larger undigested food particles and other undesirable substances such as yeast, toxins, and waste flow freely into the bloodstream, bypassing the body's normal filtering mechanisms.

You might wonder how the digestive system relates to your eczema. Simply put, the digestive system is damaged. Food enters the digestive tract and isn't properly digested because of the leaky gut. In other words, small undigested particles "leak" into the bloodstream. Once the undigested particles are floating around in your bloodstream, the body recognizes these as foreign particles and attempts to eliminate them. The elimination of these undigested particles appears in various locations on the body. Common areas are behind the knees, crease of the elbow, ankles and on the face.

The medical industry has defined all the different types of eczema and psoriasis to include specialized terms such as: Atopic eczema, Allergic contact dermatitis, Aerola eczema, Dyshidrotic eczema, Eczema herpeticum, Irritant contact dermatitis, Infantile seborrhoeic eczema, Nummular eczema, Adult seborrhoeic eczema, Varicose eczema, and Discoid eczema. As for psoriasis, types include Plaque Psoriasis, Guttate Psoriasis, Inverse Psoriasis, Pustular Psoriasis, and Scalp psoriasis.

If your specific eczema or psoriasis type is not listed, don't worry! The cause remains the same. Each person experiences symptoms in different areas, and itching may or may not be present.

Leaky Gut Syndrome serves as a powerful reminder of how interconnected our digestive health is with the rest of our body, including our skin. While eczema and psoriasis may manifest differently across individuals, the underlying cause stems from the same root issue—a compromised gut lining. Understanding this connection is crucial in addressing these conditions effectively. By healing the gut and restoring its natural barrier, you empower your body to stop treating undigested particles as invaders, reducing inflammation and alleviating symptoms. The journey toward vibrant health starts within, and taking steps to support your digestive system can lead to lasting freedom from skin-related discomforts.

Do You Know?

MEDICAL TERMINOLOGY FOR LEAKY GUT SYNDROME

INTESTINAL PERMEABILITY
GUT DYSBIOSIS
MICROBIOME IMBALANCE
GUT MICROBIAL DYSBIOSIS
HYPERPERMEABLE INTESTINES

Dysbiosis of the gut microbiome has been associated with gastrointestinal infections, obesity, allergies, auto-immune conditions, cognitive impairments, chronic enteropathies, and others.

5

YOUR GUT "FEELING" IS SPOT ON!

You know your body and that of your child more than any professional. This is your "gut feeling" or gut instinct. Therefore, keep in mind that certain foods tend to keep the body in an inflamed or leaky gut state. It's important to note that not every food listed below will affect everyone in the same way. These foods serve as a general guideline for eczema/psoriasis sufferers, as they often hinder any improvement in symptoms. While some foods may have been tested under the guidance of an allergist or medical doctor, it's important to acknowledge that these tests are not always accurate.

Allow me to share my personal experience with allergy testing. After undergoing RAST (radioallergosorbent test) and skin prick blood allergy tests, the nurse informed me of the results. "Your son is allergic to milk and peanuts, but he can consume as much corn as he wants." What? I never requested milk and peanuts to be tested; I already knew he had allergies to these common foods. I had requested an entirely different list of foods to be tested. To make matters worse, the nurse told me he could eat unlimited amounts of corn, which was infuriating. Just one bite of corn would trigger an instant asthma attack. How much did I pay for these tests? How much pain did my son endure for these absurd results? The nurse's response was astonishing: "Well, you know, Mrs. McShane, these test results are only 50-50 accurate." So, there you have it, these test results are not accurate.

An article in the Wall Street Journal featured an interview with Dr. Robert Wood, who deserves praise for his complete honesty regarding the accuracy of allergy tests. The article highlights that the results from various allergy tests are not always reliable.

“Are these blood tests being overused? Possibly. Misinterpreted? Absolutely,” says Robert Wood, director of Pediatric Allergy and Immunology at Johns Hopkins Hospital, who is part of a task force writing guidelines for diagnosing and managing food allergies. “A lot of these kids truly have food allergies, just not to all the foods that they are being told they have allergies to.”

(Source: https://www.midislandallergy.com/food-allergy-testing-and-diagnosis-wsj-article/)

As a parent, you know your child better than any doctor. Observe their reaction after eating and keep a food diary—it may sound laborious, but it works. Be attentive to any patterns that arise whenever a certain food is consumed.

A Food Elimination Diet is an excellent method for testing food sensitivities. (Did you notice the change in terminology from "food allergy" to "food sensitivity"? More on that later.) Better yet, the food elimination diet can be conducted in the comfort of your own home, producing fairly accurate results—and it's completely free!

How do you perform a Food Elimination Diet? You may have heard this term and it's quite simple. Some elimination diets recommend a 28-day elimination of soy, gluten, dairy, eggs, and yeast. While this is a great approach, it can be very challenging for some individuals. Since success is the goal, try eliminating one food for 7 days. On the 8th day, reintroduce the food you are currently testing by having it for breakfast, followed by another serving at 10:00 AM, and once more for lunch. If the food bothers you, your body will react in some way. You will know.

For instance, every time my son ate noodles, he would fall sound asleep within 5-10 minutes—head down, snoring, completely asleep. We found it initially amusing until we realized it was a reaction to a food. Over time, we discovered the connection between commercial noodles and mold; it was the mold on the noodles that bothered him. Yes, noodles can be moldy.

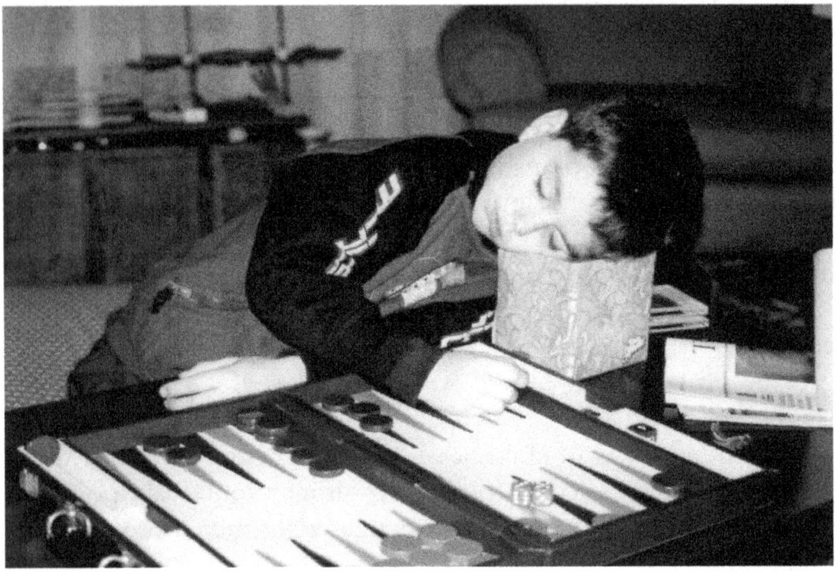

Often, individuals with eczema/psoriasis are sensitive to milk and all milk products. Start the elimination diet by removing all milk products for 7 days. These include milk, cheese, yogurt, and any food with whey or casein (a milk byproduct). On the 8th day, reintroduce milk by drinking a glassful and/or consume cheese. Pay attention to how you feel. Does your eczema flare? Look for any signs. Refer to the list of symptoms (below) to watch for, such as nose itch, rash, runny nose, gas, sneezing, watery eyes, fever, sleepiness, lethargy, cough, constipation, diarrhea, stomach pain, ringing in the ears, and swelling. The list can go on indefinitely; any symptom could be a signal that something is wrong.

After completing the milk challenge, try eliminating gluten. This might be a bit more challenging as gluten is found in various foods beyond bread and wheat products. Barley, beer, sauces, breaded foods, crackers, breakfast cereals, snack foods, soy sauce, and more contain gluten.

Once again, follow a 7-day challenge, and on the 8th day, reintroduce the food into your diet. Some clients never return to the food after just a few days because they immediately feel better or notice a reduction in eczema symptoms.

How do you choose which foods to test in an elimination diet? As mentioned earlier, start with milk and gluten. A good allergist will suggest eliminating your favorite food. It may seem counterintuitive that your body is allergic/sensitive to your favorite food, but sometimes the body can be sensitive to and crave such foods.

Here is a list of food groups to test at home:

1. Milk and all milk byproducts (check labels, whey is a milk byproduct)
2. Gluten (found in all breads, crackers, and wheat-containing sweets)
3. Eggs
4. Peanuts
5. Corn (including high fructose corn syrup)
6. Soy
7. Shellfish
8. Nightshade vegetables – potatoes, tomatoes, eggplant, and green pepper
9. Tree nuts

Here is a list of food sensitivity symptoms in adults, children and infants:

- Adults: Brain fog, fatigue, flushed skin, itching, cough, joint pain, headaches, sneezing, runny nose, bloating, gas, diarrhea, rashes, mouth ulcers, heartburn, nausea, constipation.
- Children: Red ears, flushed face, fatigue, cough, congestion, poor behavior/irritability, aggressive behavior, vomiting, stomach pain, itching, hives, swelling of lips, tongue, throat, wheezing, trouble breathing, constipation/diarrhea.
- Infants: Fussiness, crying, burping, spit up, gas, inability to sleep, rash, runny nose, red ears, cough, bloating, diarrhea, eczema, rash, itching.

Not all food reactions fit into the above categories. Food sensitivities can cause odd reactions, so it is important to remain vigilant, especially with children.

In my own experience, when my daughter was 4 years old, she used to sleepwalk and cry while going from her bedroom to the top of the stairs. We realized she was not awake during these episodes and decided to keep a detailed diary of her food intake. It became apparent that every time she consumed sodium nitrates (found in hot dogs, bacon and processed meats), she would sleepwalk. By eliminating sodium nitrates from her diet, we were able to eliminate sleepwalking. Interestingly, in her early 20s, she discovered that sodium nitrates were causing her recurrent cold sores.

Dr. Doris Rapp, an Environmental Pediatric Physician in Phoenix, Arizona, had a patient who discovered that tomatoes caused aggressive behavior in her child. Watch the entire show at http://www.youtube.com/watch?v=fRD

A client who was experiencing severe anxiety found that once she eliminated milk products from her diet, the anxiety symptoms disappeared.

Another client diagnosed with Multiple Sclerosis had difficulty maintaining a full-time job due to illness and downtime. We discovered that his MS symptoms would flare up every time he consumed sodium nitrates. A young teenage client experienced frequent migraine headaches, once gluten was eliminated the headaches disappeared.

In conclusion, the body can exhibit food sensitivities in various ways. It is important to keep an open mind and pay attention, especially when it comes to children, as their reactions can differ significantly from adults. Your gut instinct will be more accurate than the 50-50 RAST and allergy tests, guaranteed!

6

FOODS THAT STEAL

Healing eczema starts with healing the gut, and one of the most critical steps is identifying and eliminating foods that trigger inflammation. For many, eczema symptoms are exacerbated by specific food sensitivities—reactions that might not fit the traditional definition of allergies but are nonetheless harmful. These sensitivities can cause internal inflammation, leading to a leaky gut and worsening eczema. By understanding which foods are most likely to cause issues and making intentional dietary changes, you can create an environment in your body that supports healing and reduces flare-ups.

Allergies - Every eczema patient is at least sensitive to a food or food group. I use the term "allergy" cautiously as it has a well-defined meaning. Allergy is defined as "any adverse reaction to food in which the immune system is demonstrably involved. This usually requires laboratory testing to identify the IgE antibody reaction, which is considered a true food allergy." (Source: Allergies Disease in Disguise)

When discussing allergies with your doctor, they are looking for traditional allergic reactions. You may not experience those "traditional" symptoms, but you may still be reacting in other ways, such as eczema/psoriasis. From now on, I will use the term "sensitivity." In my experience, sensitivities can be equally harmful to individuals. However, the medical definition for food sensitivities is as follows:

Food sensitivity or intolerance is a reaction triggered by the digestive system. Symptoms include gas, bloating, diarrhea, constipation, cramping, and nausea. (Source: Healthline https://www.healthline.com/health/allergies/food-allergy-sensitivity-difference)

Food intolerance and sensitivity are often used interchangeably, and in some cases, it may refer to a food allergy. Regardless, the food should be avoided.

First, we need to eliminate the foods that cause your body to react. Here is a list of foods commonly found to aggravate eczema sufferers, causing internal inflammation and a leaky gut. These are the foods that inflame:

High avoidance:

High Fructose Corn Syrup (HFCS) – Eliminate 100% from your diet, this is a super toxin to your body. Contrary to the claim made by the Corn Refiners Association that there is no difference between sugar and HFCS, Dr. Mark Hyman's research indicates otherwise. HFCS, in high doses, has been shown to damage the intestinal lining, allowing harmful byproducts of gut bacteria and partially digested food proteins to enter the bloodstream and trigger inflammation, which is known to be the root cause of various health issues. Naturally occurring fructose in fruit, which is part of a complex of nutrients and fiber, does not exhibit the same biological effects as the high fructose doses found in corn sugar. (Source: Dr. Hyman's blog http://drhyman.com/blog/conditions/5-reasons-high-fructose-corn-syrup-will-kill-you/)

Gatorade, sodas, pancake syrup, and most sugary snack foods contain HFCS. Even a small amount can trigger a skin flare-up for eczema/psoriasis sufferers. Be very careful when reading food labels, below is a list of the current different names for HFCS.

1. Maize syrup
2. Glucose syrup
3. Glucose-fructose syrup
4. Fruit fructose
5. Crystalline fructose
6. High Fructose Corn Syrup
7. Isoglucose
8. Corn syrup
9. Dahlia syrup

Refined Sugar - Refined sugar is a highly processed food. The original sugar ("raw" sugar) has all the essential elements removed, resulting in a pure white final product. Since all the impurities (nutrients) have been stripped, table sugar does not require digestion. Refined sugar not only causes blood sugar swings but also promotes the growth of harmful bacteria in the digestive tract, leading to inflammation and leaky gut syndrome. Eczema sufferers should minimize their consumption of refined sugar. Switch to real maple syrup, honey or coconut sugar all these foods contain essential minerals that do not cause the same digestive issues as refined sugar.

Milk and all milk products - This may not apply to everyone, but a significant number of eczema/psoriasis sufferers cannot tolerate milk products. See "How to do an Elimination Diet" to test if you are sensitive to milk products. Interestingly, raw milk can have a healing effect as it retains naturally occurring enzymes that are destroyed during the pasteurization process. For example, those who are lactose intolerant may find it easier to digest or "tolerate" lactose in raw milk due to the presence of the enzyme lactase, which aids in lactose breakdown.

Just like High Fructose Corn Syrup, milk can be found in many products but not listed as "milk". For example, casein and whey are milk by products. A full list of milk products and alternative terms can be found at the Kids with Food Allergies website: https://community.kidswithfoodallergies.org/blog/hidden-names-for-milk-on-labels-avoidance-list-for-milk-allergy

My daughter was violently allergic to milk and milk products as a child. She has avoided milk products ever since. She now lives in Washington state where raw milk is sold in the grocery stores. She has been happily consuming raw milk and raw milk products (cheese and homemade yogurt) with no digestive issues. This is very common, pasteurized milk is very difficult to digest since all the digestive enzymes were destroyed in the processing. Have you ever noticed that pasteurized milk must have vitamin A & D added? This is synthetic vitamin A & D, you are being robbed of the real vitamins! To find raw milk in your area, visit this terrific resource: https://www.realmilk.com/raw-milk-finder/

Processed foods - breakfast cereals, candy bars, candy, soda, sports drinks, baked goods, microwave dinners. The rule of thumb is, if you must read a label, then don't eat it.

Commercially raised beef and chicken – These poor crowded animals are mistreated, placed in high stress environments, lack sunshine and consume food that is loaded with pesticides and are genetically modified. The result is sick animals that require antibiotics, tetracycline, and vaccines to keep them alive (sound familiar?). The resulting meat the eczema sufferer consumes contains all the toxins from pesticides, antibiotics and genetically modified foods. In other words, this toxic meat is inhibiting the human body from properly recovering and thriving.

My son was allergic to all meats except the lamb we obtained from a local farmer. It never occurred to me it was the toxins in the commercially raised beef and chicken that was inhibiting his ability to consume these foods. I should have figured this out on my own, especially since he could eat venison. Both the lamb and venison were "organic" since the animals had clean diets.

Choose locally sourced meats that are "regeneratively" raised. Visit local farmers markets and ask. Do you feed your animals GMO corn, use antibiotics and tetracycline? Consuming properly, humanely raised animals will make a huge difference in recovery.

> **Concentrated Animal Feeding Operations (CAFO)**
>
> **Commercially raised animals are subjected to confinement to consume pesticide covered grain diets. Obviously not their natural foods or movement. These animals become sick requiring antibiotics.**
>
> **Organically Grown Animals**
>
> **Organically Gown Animals - Farmer must adhere to a strict set of standards, must pay for certification. A better option than commercially grown meats.**
>
> **Regeneratively Raised Animals**
>
> **Farmer focuses on soil health, biodiversity, avoids synthetic pesticides and fertilizers. Enriches the soil by rotating the animals and crops. Animals roam freely, naturally regenerating the soil with urine and feces. Results in nutrient dense meats. Animals have higher Omega 3 fats by large margins. Regeneratively raised animals have resiliant health due to a stressless environment, ability to move and eat.**
>
> **Good Energy - Casey Means, M.D.**

Peanuts – It is very unusual to find an eczema/psoriasis sufferer that can tolerate peanuts. Unlike tree nuts, peanuts are grown in the ground. Therefore, peanuts tend to hold on to mold more readily than other food groups. It is the mold that affects the eczema sufferer.

Medium avoidance:

Nightshade vegetables – potatoes, tomatoes, eggplant, and green pepper

Non-organic animal meats (due to the anti-biotics)

Foods with pesticides (non-organic) – concentrate on organic fruits and vegetables

Food dyes, food additives, food preservatives

Wheat products

Shellfish

Soy

Eggs

Low Avoidance:

Fruit juices

Tree nuts

Taking control of your diet is one of the most powerful steps you can take toward healing your gut and reducing eczema symptoms. By eliminating high-risk foods like high fructose corn syrup, refined sugar, processed foods, and certain animal products, and by opting for clean, organic, and minimally processed alternatives, you give your body the best chance to repair itself from within. Be patient, listen to your body, and make adjustments as needed. With time and commitment, the foods you choose to eat can become a source of nourishment and healing rather than a trigger for discomfort.

7

FOODS THAT HEAL

Healing your digestive tract doesn't have to feel overwhelming—it can actually be an enjoyable and rewarding process. Start by assessing your current diet. Make a list of the foods you typically eat over the course of a week and compare it to the "Foods that Steal" list discussed earlier. Do you notice any potential connections between your dietary choices and persistent digestive inflammation? The good news is that shifting your focus to nutrient-rich, gut-healing foods can not only soothe your symptoms but also set the foundation for long-term health. By embracing foods that nourish and repair, you're taking a powerful step toward healing from the inside out.

Foods that heal:

1. Foods high in Omega-3
2. Fermented foods
3. Fruits and vegetables
4. Bone broth (just like Great Grandma used to make)

1 - Foods High in Omega-3s

Fish - Salmon is an excellent source but be cautious about its origin. Limit farmed salmon to once a month and opt for wild-caught salmon. Farmed fish are often given antibiotics, chlorine, and other toxins due to their crowded conditions. Canned herring or kippers are also high in Omega-3 and delicious when paired with mayonnaise on a cracker.

Chia seeds - These little powerhouses have become popular due to their portability, high nutritional value, easy storage, and abundant Omega-3 content. They are favored by serious athletes, food enthusiasts, nutritionists, and even eczema sufferers. A small amount goes a long way in helping to heal the digestive tract and simultaneously providing great energy. You can find chia seeds at most health food stores and some specialty grocery retailers like Wegmans and Whole Foods.

Cod Liver Oil – This is the best supplement to consume to heal the digestive system. Grandmother was a fan of cod liver oil for a good reason. It is an excellent source of Omega 3, reduces internal inflammation and is a natural source of vitamins A & D. Supplement vendors offer palatable options for young children (and us adults!).

2 - Fermented foods

Sadly, this category of food has been missing from the American diet for many years. Probably one of the most important keys to healing the digestive track. I know you are thinking, but I eat yogurt every day, doesn't that count? Yes and no. Yogurt products are typically made from pasteurized and homogenized milk then sugar is added. Between the pasteurized milk (which allergy sufferers typically cannot tolerate) and the sugar, most benefit from the yogurt is erased. Making your own raw milk yogurt is within reach if your state allows the sale of raw milk. Currently, many states are under pressure to offer raw milk, Pennsylvania and Washington offer raw milk at boutique grocery stores. France has always offered raw milk, even in vending machines. Look to see if your state offers raw milk: https://www.realmilk.com/raw-milk-finder/

Raw Sauerkraut – You can make your own inexpensively, however raw sauerkraut can be purchased at the health food store. Do not heat the sauerkraut, eat it as is. This food is loaded with the full spectrum of probiotics that will assist in healing the digestive track.

Kefir - Unfortunately, commercially available kefir is typically made with pasteurized milk. However, kefir seeds are available for purchase, and you can easily make coconut kefir at home using coconut milk. There are also a few commercial coconut kefir products on the market, although they are just starting to become available.

Kombucha - This delicious drink is easy to make at home and far better than most commercial varieties. Commercial kombucha must be pasteurized which erases many of the valuable probiotics. Enjoy a glass of homemade kombucha before your evening meal, it's very similar to a glass of wine!

3 – Fruits and Vegetables

Fruits - Whenever possible, opt for organic fruits to avoid pesticides. If certain fruits are not in season, check out the frozen section of your grocery store. Frozen fruits like blueberries, strawberries, "smoothie" fruits, peaches, and pineapple are "fresh" frozen and may have a higher vitamin content compared to fruits that have been in transit for weeks. Stock up on various fruits and toss them in the freezer for easy access.

Vegetables - fresh and locally grown options are best. However, when they're not available, frozen organic vegetables serve as a good alternative. Leafy greens are an excellent source of vitamins, making them ideal for a "Healing Smoothie" recipe that should be incorporated into your daily routine. Starting your day with a healthy breakfast and a smoothie ensures you include the three key foods for healing your eczema in your diet every day. If you're short on time, you can prepare the ingredients in the blender the night before. In the morning, simply blend and pour the contents into a mason jar that can be taken with you and consumed throughout the day.

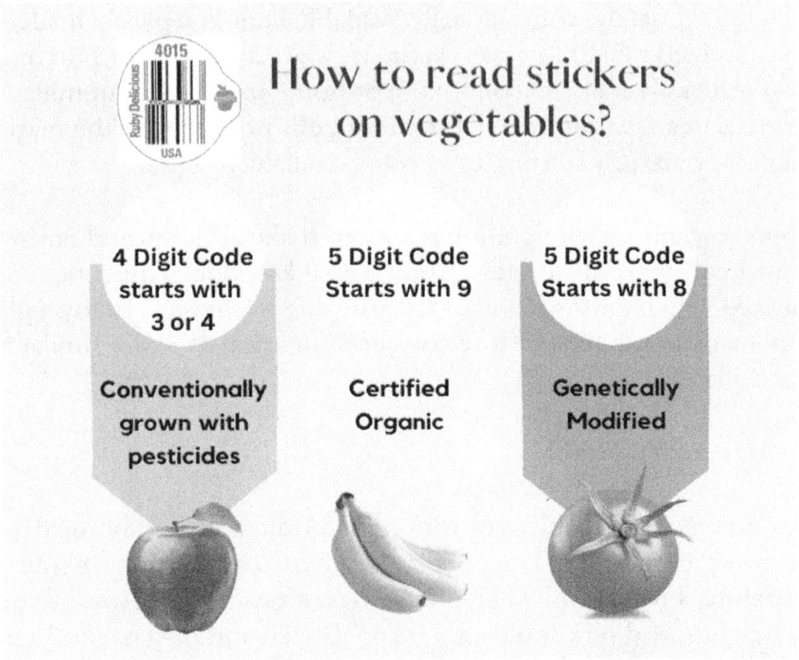

4 - Bone Broth

This is hands down, the magic gut healing food. Investing in an Instant Pot will make your life easier. After making two rounds of bone broth, you will have already made up for the investment. A quart of bone broth typically sells for $10, so if you're currently discarding organic chicken, beef, or any animal bones, you're missing out on a nutrient-dense healing food. Making bone broth with an Instant Pot is super easy and takes just minutes, as the machine does all the work. The addition of apple cider vinegar to the water when preparing bone broth is crucial. Its purpose is to leach the minerals from the bones, remember minerals remain stable and cannot be destroyed by heat. Consuming bone broth provides a full spectrum of minerals, along with the added benefits of collagen, enzymes and amino acids. These minerals and enzymes coat the digestive tract, facilitating the healing process. The Weston Price Foundation offers blogs, podcasts, and a book that explains all the benefits of consuming bone broth.

For more information, visit:

- Weston Price Foundation blog and podcast: https://www.westonaprice.org/podcast/dont-throw-away-bones/#gsc.tab=0
- Book: Nourishing Broth: An Old-Fashioned Remedy for the Modern World

Not interested in making your own bone broth? Fair enough, I understand, and there are easy alternatives to making and consuming your own bone broth. Companies like Ancient Nutrition, Paleovalley, Left Coast Performance, and Paradise Naturals all offer a full line of bone broth powders. These powders can be mixed with coconut water, nut milks, or water to provide a quick and delicious way to consume bone broth and reap the rewards of healing the digestive tract. You can use these powders to make a superfood smoothie to supplement breakfast, lunch, or as a mid-day snack. Add fruits and/or greens to your smoothie; it's a fantastic way to heal yourself while consuming healthy food.

Liquid varieties of bone broth exist on the grocery store shelves. I do not recommend bone broth from commercially raised animals, organic sources only.

Special Mention! Collagen – A Hidden Secret to Clear Skin

Want to see immediate results from making a change? Collagen powder (a bone broth by product) is my go-to to help those who are timid about making dietary changes. Collagen powder is a super food for those with leaky gut. The powder mixed with water is tasteless and easy to drink. Its healing properties address the layer of damaged loose connective tissues that line the digestive track. As described by Dr. Josh Axe in his book, The Collagen Diet "the gut-skin connection theorizes that intestinal permeability can cause common skin conditions, including acne and psoriasis."

Purchase collagen powder from the same companies as listed above for bone broth.

8

SUPPLEMENTS FOR ECZEMA SUFFERERS

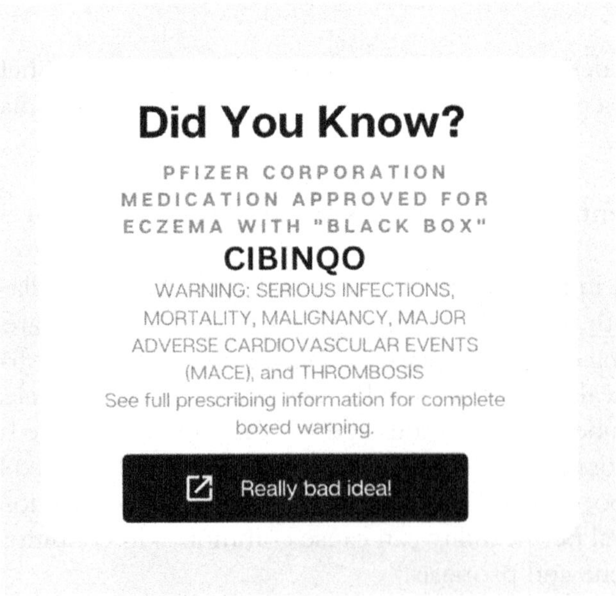

"I just want to take a pill and make the eczema go away." Think on this, a pill that does not address the source of the problem and can cause mortality?

In the late 1990's after my son was born, the internet was just starting to explode with information. At that time, there were Yahoo "discussion groups" where people could communicate worldwide, share information and bypass organized groups and professionals. I joined a Yahoo discussion group to search for answers for eczema, its causes and solutions or successes from others. In the end I was dismayed, over 90% of the subscribers were ultimately looking for a pill. Diet was not an area of interest and digestive issues were rarely discussed.

I understand the desire to find a quick solution and make eczema disappear with a pill. However, it's important to recognize that supplements can be a whole lot more beneficial for eczema sufferers than a magical pharmaceutical pill with horrendous side effects. I highly recommend healing your gut by adopting a nutrient-dense diet alongside a good vitamin regimen. Combining these two approaches will lead to faster recovery and long-term relief from eczema symptoms. The duration of the healing process depends on factors such as the severity of the condition, the health of your digestive system, and your age. Older adults may take longer to recover compared to younger adults, while children and babies tend to heal more quickly due to their resilient bodies.

How long will it take to see improvements? Most individuals will notice an improvement in their symptoms within two weeks of eliminating trigger foods, incorporating healing foods, and taking recommended supplements simultaneously. However, complete healing may take longer, possibly several years for some adults. Babies, on the other hand, can experience healing within 3-4 weeks.

It's important to remember that the healing time varies for each person, as different factors influence the process. For instance, I once had a 9-month-old client who wasn't healing as rapidly as expected. We discovered that environmental issues, specifically a moldy rented apartment, was hindering the baby's recovery. Once they relocated to a moldy free environment the baby's eczema completely cleared up.

Get serious about healing yourself, below are supplement charts for different age brackets. Do NOT skip this step in your healing process.

Essential Fatty Acids

Age	Essential Fatty Acids	Dosing
Infants 3-12 months	Green Pasture Fermented Cod Liver Oil Or Baby DHA by Nordic Naturals	1/8 Teaspoon/Dropper Follow weight instruction on package
Toddler Ages 1-6 years	Green Pasture Fermented Cod Liver Oil Or Children's DHA by Nordic Naturals	1/8 - 1/2 Teaspoon Follow weight instructions on package
Children 6-12 years	Green Pasture Fermented Cod Liver Oil Or Ultimate Omega Junior by Nordic Naturals	Follow weight instructions on package
Teens - Adults	Green Pasture Fermented Cod Liver Oil Or Ultimate Omega 2x by Nordic Naturals	Follow weight instructions on package
Picky Eaters	Barlean's Omega 3	Sweet taste, creamy texture and many varieties for the picky eater. Available at most health food stores and The Vitamin Shoppe

Note: Adults, if taking capsules, once in the morning, once in the evening to spread the healing. For infants and babies another option is to apply cod liver oil to the skin, the oil absorbs very well using this method. Apply during a diaper change, in days past most diaper rash ointment contained cod liver oil!

A highly recommended source for moms worldwide is the book, "The Nourishing Traditions Book of Baby and Child Care" by Sally Fallon Morell and Thomas S. Cowan, MD. Nutrition, recipes, product recommendations and childcare tips are carefully explained within the 300 pages of this must have book.

Probiotics

Age Bracket	Probiotic Options	Dosing
Infants 0-12 months	Mommy Bliss Or Metagenics	Follow weight instruction on package
Toddler and Children Ages 1-13 years	Mary Ruth's Dr. Formulated Organic Kids+ Natures Plus Animal Parade	Follow weight instructions on package
Teens 14-18 years	Mary Ruth Gummies Or ProBioCare	Follow weight instructions on package
Adults	Garden of Eden Dr. Formulated Renew Life	Follow dosing instructions on label

Add these daily supplements too!

Daily multi-vitamin

L-Glutamine – Stimulates intestinal mucosa growth, important amino acid to add to your healing journey

Vitamin D (Not necessary if taking Cod Liver Oil)

Zinc

Collagen

Final note, the goal is to coat the digestive track. Using supplements, bone broth, collagen, L-Glutamine and cod liver oil will speed your recovery.

Healing the digestive tract is a journey, but it's one that offers lasting rewards. By incorporating gut-nurturing foods like Omega-3-rich salmon and chia seeds, fermented foods such as kefir and raw sauerkraut, vibrant fruits and vegetables, and the timeless magic of bone broth, you're equipping your body with the tools it needs to recover and thrive. Supplements like collagen, probiotics, and cod liver oil can complement these dietary changes, accelerating the healing process.

Patience and consistency are key; while many notice improvements within weeks, full recovery may take longer. Remember, this journey is deeply personal, and external factors like environment can also play a role. Listen to your body, make adjustments as needed, and trust in the power of whole, healing foods. With commitment and care, you can transform your diet into a source of vitality and strength, paving the way for a healthier, eczema-free future.

9

ENVIRONMENTAL FACTORS

When it comes to managing eczema, environmental factors often play a more significant role than we realize. While air pollution may seem beyond our control, there are many other toxic exposures that can directly impact eczema sufferers—and these are within our power to address. Beyond the food we consume, toxins enter our bodies through three primary pathways: the mouth, the lungs, and the skin. By understanding and reducing exposure to these environmental triggers, you can create a cleaner, healthier environment that supports your healing journey.

> **Synthetic Chemicals and Environmental Toxins**
>
> **Since World War II, over 80,000 synthetic chemicals have entered our environment and approximately fifteen hundred new chemicals are released each year, many of which have never been tested for safety in adults, children or fetuses.**
>
> **..These chemicals are drivers of all three hallmarks of Bad Energy; oxidative stress, inflammation and mitochondrial dysfunction-and the link is now so sell defined that many of these chamicals are being classified as obesogens, meaning that they are known to impair metabolism in such a way that they causatively contribute to obesity and insulin resistance.**
>
> **Good Energy - Casey Means, M.D.**
> **Page 227-228**

Lungs - Reducing Airborne Toxins

Laundry detergent and fabric softeners - The fragrances (parfums) used in most commercial laundry detergents irritate individuals with eczema. The fragrances add to the sufferer's daily toxin load. Body heat and sweat cause the parfums from the laundry detergent to generate toxic fumes. The solution is simple, use fragrance-free detergent and fabric softener! However, you will need to eliminate the scent from your clothes, wash them multiple times using baking soda and white distilled vinegar. After 5-6 washes, the toxic fragrances will be greatly reduced. Switch immediately to fragrance free laundry detergent and dryer sheets. These products are referred to as "Free & Clear", free and clear of fragrances, dyes and harsh chemicals.

An environmentally friendly option is soap nuts, no plastic containers, no chemicals and very inexpensive. CURE with PURE is available through Amazon, one bag will last for over 180 loads of wash.

Aerosol sprays - Products like Windex, Lysol, furniture polish, flea and tick sprays, or any other airborne particle can affect individuals with eczema. Minimize exposure to these products as much as possible. An easy inexpensive alternative is distilled vinegar and water in a spray bottle.

New car interior, cigar, and cigarette smoke, perfumes, cosmetics, shampoos, and conditioners with potent fragrances (listed as "parfums" in the ingredient list).

Avoid new carpets, new construction, and paint fumes. Nowadays, paint companies offer paints with significantly reduced toxic fumes due to allergies. If requested in advance, carpet companies can "air out" your new carpet and padding for up to 5 weeks prior to installation.

Products that should be strictly avoided by eczema sufferers include Febreze air fresheners, Febreze sprays, scented air freshers, scented candles and dish washer detergents with a “scent”. Actively avoid perfumed garbage can liners and dish washer detergent perfumed with “fresh” or “lemon” scent. All these lingering scents and parfums cause the eczema sufferer more issues.

Pets like cats, birds, horses, and sometimes even the family dog can trigger issues for some individuals. Feathered pillows, bed covers, wool blankets, or synthetic bedding have been known to cause problems.

Simple holiday or seasonal exposures will also cause issues, real Christmas trees are often sprayed with pine scent. This factoid took us years to learn, my poor son was sick every December right after the tree was set up. Avoid the holiday scented candles and pinecones (cinnamon scent) that come along with the holiday spirit. In the summertime, be aware of pool chlorine, and many times mulch can also be problematic.

In the fall, mold can exacerbate asthma, increase allergies, and worsen eczema symptoms. As the tree leaves change colors, the leaves will often release mold spores. In your home, a simple $10.00 home testing mold kit is available at Home Depot. I had a 10-month-old client whose diet had been changed, and the environment cleaned up, but we couldn't figure out the final piece of the puzzle. A quick mold test revealed the apartment was moldy, and once the family moved the eczema disappeared.

10

SKIN TOXIN EXPOSURE

The skin acts as a vast sponge, absorbing various toxins from the air (such as laundry detergent toxins). It's important to also consider the products applied directly to the skin. Limit the use of cosmetics and hair dyes. Pay attention to the ingredients and the amount of toxins listed on the label of your shampoo, conditioner, creams and deodorants. Dry skin can be problematic but opt for creams with minimal chemicals and natural lubricants like coconut oil, shea butter or olive oil.

Hair dye is absorbed through the scalp, pregnant women are advised to avoid dying their hair to avoid toxic exposure for the fetus.

Sunblock – stay away from all sun block products! These are unsafe for eczema sufferers due to the abundance of toxins in their ingredients. Doubt that statement? Pick up the book "Sunscreens Biohazard 2: Proof of Toxicity Keeps Piling Up" by Elizabeth Plourde and Marcus Plourde, both of whom are medical research scientists. Once you read how dangerous sunblock is to our health and that of the environment, you will never use it again.

While skin professionals often recommend Vaseline, I believe it does more harm than good and do not recommend this course of action. After following the doctor's orders for my son, he suffered his worst night ever. Vaseline closes the pores, making it difficult for the body to release the undigested toxins that are the root cause of eczema.

Good Environmental Exposures

Sunshine – Exposing yourself to the sun for 15-20 minutes every day provides a good dose of vitamin D. It can also be soothing for some eczema sufferers to expose their skin to the sun. Why not give it a try?

Ocean water – The ocean is rich in minerals, and exposing your skin to sea water can be incredibly healing. A client of mine with a small child went to the beach and applied sea water to the child's skin, and the results were truly amazing!

Not near the ocean? Baja Gold Sea Salt offers a product that contains 90 essential elements harvested near a deep-sea thermal. The exciting part of their product is not only the purity of the sea salt (mined from the Baja of Mexico) but the high level of essential elements. Their newly released product Ocean Mineral Soak will soothe eczema sufferers by immersing their skin in bathwater that contains all the essential elements from sea water. https://bajagoldsaltco.com/products/ocean-mineral-soak?variant=45924397547830 Order the sea salt at the same time, you will be amazed at how great tasting sea salt can be!

Healing eczema can often be more than just dietary adjustments and require environmental toxin awareness. Environmental changes like switching to fragrance-free laundry detergents, avoiding aerosol sprays, and using natural alternatives for skin care and cleaning, you can minimize your daily toxin load. Simple yet powerful practices such as spending time in the sun, enjoying ocean water, or using mineral-rich products like Baja Gold Ocean Mineral Soak can provide additional relief and promote healing.

Remember, small, consistent changes in your environment can lead to big improvements in your skin health.

11

MEDICATIONS AND ALTERNATIVE PRACTITIONERS

My journey to find answers for my son's condition took me to various healers and practitioners. I sought help from renowned allergists, dermatologists, and pediatricians along the east coast. Then, I explored alternative care professionals, where I discovered remarkable healers and supportive caregivers. Chiropractic doctors offered valuable advice on health and nutrition. Acupuncture, a refined science of over 500 years, proved to be a fantastic alternative. It was through acupuncture professionals that I learned about NAET - Nambrudripad Allergy Elimination Technique.

NAET combines acupuncture knowledge with kinesiology to test and clear allergic reactions from the body. While this technique doesn't work for everyone, I was fortunate it worked for my son. When we began the sessions, he could only tolerate 10 foods, but after two months, his food variety doubled to 20 items. It helped improve his condition greatly. That said, there were still other aspects to address.

Homeopathy holds promises for treating eczema, although I personally haven't had experience using it for long-term chronic illnesses. This doesn't mean it won't work, but during the mid-1990s, a homeopathic and medical doctor I worked with did not offer a solution for eczema using homeopathic medicines. This is not my area of expertise or experience and is not covered further in this book. Times may have changed, so it could be worth exploring.

Medications have their benefits and have saved my son's life on many occasions. However, I didn't want him to rely on medications indefinitely. As a baby, we used Benadryl to alleviate his pain, and later, occasional asthma medication. Over time, individuals with a leaky gut can become allergic or sensitive to their medications. If you suspect that the medication is doing more harm than good, it's important to discuss this with your doctor.

12

SUMMARY

I wish I had known then what I know now. If only I had this book to read 20 years ago, it would have spared my son numerous doctor visits and emergency trips to the hospital. My goal is to spread the word that healing from eczema is possible. You don't have to live with it or believe the common notion that its cause is unknown and there is no cure.

The cure lies within these pages.

1. Eliminate all processed foods.
2. Consume a diet rich in Omega 3s.
3. Opt for organic meats, fruits and vegetables.
4. Incorporate fermented foods into your daily routine.
5. Drink bone broth every day.
6. Take the recommended supplements.
7. Exercise, get fresh air, and sunshine.

Thank you for reading this book, may God bless you with health, happiness, and clear skin forever!

13

RECIPES

Time to take a break and grab a healthy snack! Start with an easy quick snack, high in Omega3, healthy fats and inexpensive.

Canned Smoked Kippers

Add mayonnaise (made with avocado oil) and eat with rice crackers. For those who are more adventurous, add jalapeno peppers.

Chia Seed Pudding

1 cup liquid (any milk will do)
4 tbsp. chia seeds
1 tsp. sweetener (raw honey or maple syrup)
1/2 tsp. vanilla
1 scoop collagen (www.ancientnutrition.com)
(Add fresh berries, banana or other fruit)
Add all ingredients to a mason jar. Either use a frother or stir to blend evenly. Set in refrigerator for 2 hours or over night.

Gut Healing Smoothie

1 scoop Bone Broth Protein Powder (www.ancientnutrition.com)
Coconut water
Banana

1 scoop collagen
Add ingredients to a blender and enjoy!

Cherry Vanilla Collagen Smoothie

1 1/2 cup coconut milk
1 cup frozen cherries
1 scoop vanilla Bone Broth Protein powder (www.ancientnutrition.com)
1 scoop collagen (www.ancientnutrition.com)
Ice cubes (optional)
Place ingredients in a blender, blend until smooth.

Collagen Coffee

1 ½ cups organic brewed coffee
1 tablespoon butter from grass fed cows
1 tablespoon coconut oil
1 scoop collagen
1 scoop vanilla Bone Broth Protein powder (optional)
Place in a blender, blend until smooth.

Homemade Bone Broth Recipe

Two options, cook on the stovetop for 24 hours at a simmer or cook in an Instant Pot for 4 hours under pressure.
Chicken bones – (roast an organic chicken, consume all the meat)
2 Carrots chopped into 1 inch pieces
2 Celery stalks chopped into 1 inch pieces
1 Onion quartered including the skin
1 tbsp. apple cider vinegar
Add enough water to completely cover the bones (4-5 quarts)
Optional – add spices, chicken feet (adds more collagen)
Place all ingredients into a pot, add vinegar and let sit for 45 minutes (extracts additional minerals from the bones). Simmer for 24 hours or under pressure for 4 hours. When completed, discard all the ingredients, pass through a metal mesh strainer into quart mason jars. Makes approximately 5 quarts. Freeze jars that may not be used immediately

14

ADDENDUM

VACCINES: ECZEMA SUFFERERS BEWARE

Atopic Dermatitis and Vaccinations Against Smallpox, Measles, Mumps and Rubella

Children and adults diagnosed with atopic dermatitis (eczema) should not receive the smallpox vaccine. According to the Centers for Disease Control and Prevention (CDC), individuals who have ever been diagnosed with atopic dermatitis, even if the condition is mild or not currently active, are at a higher risk of developing serious complications if exposed to the smallpox vaccine virus.

People with atopic dermatitis should be cautious when in close physical contact with someone who has recently received the smallpox vaccine. It is important to ensure that the vaccinated person covers the vaccination site or takes other precautions until the scab falls off (about 3 weeks).

Atopic dermatitis can be exacerbated following vaccination for measles, mumps, rubella, or measles infection. In other words, tell your doctor to wave the MMR vaccine for your child due to the severe side effects that will result from the vaccine. (Source: https://pubmed.ncbi.nlm.nih.gov/14690341/)

In my journey with my son's severe eczema, I chose to avoid all vaccines until we could understand the underlying cause. It was a challenging path to navigate, considering the medical and school pressures to vaccinate him. Thankfully, in the state of Maryland, we have the religious exemption, which I utilized by stating, "I am religiously against all vaccinations." Whenever the school nurse called, I would invite her to lunch to discuss my religious beliefs, and she never took me up on that lunch offer!

When my son went to college, the nurse insisted on mandating the meningitis vaccine. I pointed out that the vaccine mandate only applied to those pursuing medical studies. Stand your ground, as your child does not belong to the state, and you are solely responsible for their well-being. Vaccines and eczema do not mix well since vaccines introduce additional toxins into the bloodstream, which eczema sufferers cannot tolerate.

Recent news regarding post-COVID-19 vaccine effects has shed light on the dangers of the 72 mandated childhood vaccines. At one point, only 5% of the US population was vaccine non-compliant however, the numbers have been steadily increasing. In 2022 the non-compliance rate went to 10%. Parents are thankfully waking up to this issue. (Source: https://www.cdc.gov/mmwr/volumes/72/wr/mm7202a2.htm)

Robert Kennedy Jr. has been involved in litigating the side effects of the childhood vaccine schedule for over 20 years. It is crucial to educate yourself on this longstanding issue. I highly recommend listening to Joe Rogan's Spotify Podcast interview with Mr. Kennedy (first 45 minutes), as it will provide shocking insights. Please note that there are attempts to remove this interview by the censor police, so catch it before that happens. (Source: https://open.spotify.com/episode/3DQfcTY4viyXsIXQ89NXvg)

Embark on a journey of transformation to reclaim your (or your child’s) life from the clutches of eczema and psoriasis! In this well researched book, the author shares her inspiring tale of discovering gut dysbiosis as the cause of eczema. Free from the limitations of traditional medicine, she unveils a treasure trove of research, nutrition, and a no-nonsense guide that will empower you to rewrite your skin's story. This invaluable roadmap for infants, children, and adults is your passport to clear skin. Unleash the power of targeted nutrition and supplementation with carefully curated sources and age-specific dosing. Delve into a world of hope as you explore medical and non-medical resources that validate the astounding success stories of the author's health coach clients. The path to clear skin is real, it is within your reach, and it starts with this extraordinary book!

INDEX

ABOUT THE AUTHOR

Jolie McShane is a mother of three terrific children and the wife of a very supportive husband. Jolie received her Health Coach Certification in 2011 through the Institute of Integrative Nutrition. She coaches those with eczema, allergies and asthma to better health.

Jolie is not intimidated by the medical establishment due to the hours of research and education to heal her son. One doctor would even take notes during office visits! A business professional and community volunteer, Jolie is well known in the Baltimore area. This is her first book. Additional books about asthma and allergies are in the works.

Jolie's additional training courses include:

Institute for Integrative Nutrition Certified Health Coach
Blueprint for Environmental Toxins
Talking Toxins Course
IIN Gut Health Course
IIN Hormone Health Course
Liver Lovers Challenge

Made in the USA
Monee, IL
04 November 2026

67379963R00036